6 SMALL MEDITATION MEALS A DAY

BITE-SIZED MEDITATIONS TO FUEL YOUR BUSY DAY

BONNIE GRIFFIN

Copyright © 2019 by Bonnie Griffin

All rights reserved. This book may not be reproduced or stored
in whole or in part by any means without the written permission of
the author except for brief quotations for the purpose of review.

ISBN: 978-1-7338973-9-6

Edited by: Allie Coker and Monika Dziamka

Published by Warren Publishing
Charlotte, NC
www.warrenpublishing.net

Printed in the United States

*This book is dedicated with much
gratitude to Butch, for showing patience
and love throughout all my endeavors.*

TABLE OF CONTENTS

Dear Stress—

*By the time I finish reading this book,
we will not be on speaking terms.*

INTRODUCTION

The electromagnetic sensors made it hard to move my head from side to side. My arms were stiff, and my chest felt uncomfortable.

"Stay very still," the doctor emphasized for the third time. He didn't know me very well. Didn't he understand I was here because I'm a high-octane human? Of course, I'm fidgety. It goes hand in hand with being a high-energy person.

It was 1995 and biofeedback was supposed to reveal why I was having severe migraines, complicated digestive issues, and unrelenting nightmares. I laughed when I caught a glimpse of my wired self in the mirror. The doctor ran into the room during the test and asked *exactly* what I had been thinking just then. He was curious because my numbers had suddenly plummeted in the best way.

"Laughter," I explained with a smile. Thirty pages of analytical data only made this thirty-year-old feel that the answer was too complicated and a trip to the comedy club that night was all I really needed.

I was working three jobs to pay my way through graduate school. Stress was my natural companion, but I was convinced it would all go away soon enough. In the second month of starting my first business, I had added another doctor to the list. This time it was an oral surgeon to help control the severe TMJ brought on by you-know-what. By the time I was forty and started my second business, the effects of stress on the body were common knowledge and well-known to most, but we busy humans leave ourselves little choice other than to keep running toward the goal and hoping for the best. God knows there is no one else who can do the job we do. We accept the stress as obligatory—it's part of the process of being who we are, after all. We find ways to relieve the stress we accumulate instead of eliminating the source of the problem.

I didn't ask for the pills the doctor gave me for headaches and severe jaw pain. We work long, hard hours all day, so a little help can't hurt. Most of my colleagues enjoy a routine wind-down drink after work before starting all over again the next day. By business number three, the larger stressors began to pile on top of smaller mounds of stress. Business associates my age were having heart attacks, and vacation became a saving grace, a must-do, and the only time I was free from the physical pangs. It began to go something like this: *stress … stress … VACATION … less stress … stress.* As an entrepreneur working seven days a week, vacation was my *only* break. A former nine-to-five job with weekends off allowed for some respite, but then Sunday night came the dread.

I've seen other entrepreneurs get pushed so far on the stress scale that they approach a breaking point, and you can almost see them reaching for a cleaver to sever the cord of tension in one whack. I know I'm overly stressed when homesteading in the Alaskan wilderness starts to sound appealing to this southern sorority girl. Although those who boldly go "off the grid" are extreme cases in our minds, they do demonstrate an appealing element of wanting to break free.

We, the more practical, simply call going off the grid another vacation and, for many, the vacations become more frequent. A pattern emerges that we are all too familiar with—relax on vacation, and the stress begins again the moment you pull back into your driveway of reality. The giant (expensive) Band-Aid we put on our problem has just been ripped off with little-to-no warning. Welcome home.

I began to wonder: what would happen if we could bring the vacation home with us? Not just the souvenir shell and the t-shirt proclaiming, "I ate the whole burger," but the primary elements—the feelings, the attitude, the relaxation of the body. What if we could somehow bring these things into our daily lives? Wouldn't it be great to have a clear, creative mind on a Tuesday and not just in the tropics? We feel our bodies creeping back to old patterns of stress two days before hotel check-out. How great would it be to feel okay with going back to the necessary routine of work?

Busy people are good at creating success for themselves but don't slow down on their own very well, and more success means more stress. This, in turn, means less time to get away; however, when you do take the time, the vacations tend to be more elaborate and more expensive. That's great (good for you), but it doesn't help the cynical cycle of stress.

Mergers and Migraines

I had left the house in plenty of time to arrive at the convention center, but the blinding pain over my left eye made driving difficult. Speaking to a crowd of one hundred wasn't the cause. I had prepared my speech well, and the crowd was sure to be an agreeable one. They say migraines show up between twenty-four to forty-eight hours after a major stressor, which is often unidentifiable. I ran the calendar backward in my hurting head as if it even mattered. I was ten minutes ahead of schedule, which allowed me to make a quick stop. Ice for the head, a shot of caffeine, and a prayer I could make it through the thirty-minute talk without them noticing my pain.

On top of pain comes the frustration of knowing you are smiling less, lacking in inspiration, and just not at your best. Those of us who are very motivated, high energy, and Type A tell ourselves we will deal with pain at the end of the day. We squeeze in a salad at lunch to make us feel like we are doing something right to address the stress, but the unpredictability of stress-induced illnesses makes looking forward to special events a challenge to say the least. We may love the work we do; we love our friends and hobbies, but the road to that enjoyment can be intense and unwavering as if there is a high price to pay for being who we are. I would eventually figure out how to slash those high prices, but in the meantime another vacation would have to suffice. I headed to the spas of Arizona.

The Spa Within You

The healing hands of a stranger greeted me in my plastic flip-flops and oversized robe. The gentle laps of ocean waves played in the background. I had worked hard all year to get to that relaxing environment in central Arizona. I was once again soothed but not satisfied as the inevitable return to stress loomed like a dark cloud in the dim room.

"Try to relax and don't think about work," the voice beside me said. Her hands eased the words across my back. I drifted off thinking about those who experience way more stress than I ever will, yet they find a way to rise above, function, and juggle without caving in like many newsworthy celebs have done. What about those who don't like their jobs or love their jobs and can't stand their bosses? I love what I do—so why am I having chest pains?

To bring these two worlds of peace and work together would mean creative, clear generation of new practices during the workday and not just miles away once or twice a year. What if the spa existed within us all? Thousands of dollars are spent to manufacture something that is within our possession anytime, anywhere no matter what the circumstance.

As I warmed my toes by the fireplace on day two of my Arizona adventure, the questions still circled in my mind. *I have control over several business and I've always known what to do to get to where I am today. Why then can't I take control over the stress with the same skill and dedication that allowed me this vacation?* We are all born with an inner fortitude and ability to coach ourselves, yet many of us do not look for it within ourselves. Instead, we search for these qualities externally. We turn to physical comforts such as alcohol, medications, a more organized assistant, or a relationship that helps us forget the stress for a while. I knew in that moment in Arizona that my vacation would not end *this* time when I stepped off the plane back home.

SIX MEDS ARE
BETTER THAN ONE

The seed was planted as I headed back east from Arizona. Vacations are great, don't get me wrong, but I needed to gain control of the home-front, and I knew I would start with the popular morning meditation. The concept was new to me yet not unfamiliar. I ordered a CD, made a comfortable spot in my den, and began to breathe in slowly. Seven seconds later, I exhaled. During my first few 6 a.m. attempts at meditation, my mind wandered—an obvious expectation for a brain full of to-do lists and exploding Mind Maps. As I sat in silence, my mind drifted back to the year 2002.

I was seated in the waiting room of my family doctor ready for round three of the blood tests. Drastically dropping down the energy ladder every afternoon was not aiding in my climb to the top. Once again, a doctor was surprised and threw a door open.

"I've never seen levels this low," he said. That's when I faded out. In the recovery room, I was instructed to consider eating several mini-meals throughout the day, which was not a strange concept. I had heard of many others praising this routine. Eating on-the-go would actually be a better fit for me.

I snapped back to my dimly lit den hoping my kids would stay asleep for a few more minutes. I tried not to be mad at myself for the constant mental drifting. I knew this was part of training the brain to focus and that, as a person with a never-quiet brain, any progress was admirable. Breathe in, breathe out, and five minutes later I was already feeling better and ready to take on my day. Meditation was working!

By 9:30 a.m., my coffee and morning meditation were gone. Staff meetings, starred emails, unrealistic to-do lists, and electrical problems from last night's storm replaced any sense of peace I had achieved. Did I mention it was only 9:30 a.m.?

For the busy human, life is a constant pull of decision-making, financial ups and downs, and unrelenting obligations to keep things rolling. I grabbed one of my snacks as I walked into the staff meeting knowing that what I really needed was another meditation—but that would have to wait until tomorrow morning, right? Thus, I began my search for more than the morning meditation, something that could carry me through the day emotionally the way six little meals can do physically.

So many times, we start the workday with a positive, calm attitude and a spark in our eye. Then something gets thrown at us, making us wonder where the peaceful feeling went, and we often feel guilty for not being able to maintain the level of positivity throughout the day. An outburst at a coworker may take us by surprise. I love my work, so why am I so stressed? We have no idea what triggers the frustration, the outbursts, and the anger. All we know is how to plan the next getaway (or make some great weekend plans) when what we really need is a more permanent solution.

Most people find peace early in the day as they grip their morning cup of calm and unwind at night, but in between, chaos develops. The purpose of this book is to demolish that chaos and bring the vacation home. I am certain that in doing so, you will be more productive, create more success, and erase the dread of Sunday night or the end of your week in the tropics. What I didn't expect for myself was how quickly the stress-related illnesses would begin to disappear—no more frequent trips to the doctor, no more medications, no migraines or chest pains, and no more nightmares!

Six Small Meditation Meals a Day seeks to give power to your moments and peace where there was once chaos. It replaces the time wasted on stress with new ideas. These mini-meditation meals break up your day into manageable segments with a unique focus for each area. The program allows for flexibility, and the six meditations are easily incorporated into meditation apps with habit reminders and pleasing notifications. Think of it as meditation on-the-go. You're taking back your day in a meditative way with a new focus every couple of hours.

Six Small Meditation Meals a Day can be modified to fit your schedule, but I suggest two in the morning, two in the afternoon, and two in the evening. Think you are too busy to pause? Any of the six mini-meditations can be a walking meditation or practiced in the silence of a bathroom stall. The key component is to stop and react to your moment of focus. Smile, pause, and slow down long enough to let the universe do its work on you. Have you ever tried to take a splinter out of a kid's finger? They squirm and scream not realizing that being calm gets them the help they need. The universe needs you to be in pause mode to inspire you and, in exchange for a few minutes a day, the way you react to stress will be drastically transformed.

With *Six Small Meditation Meals a Day,* you will quickly begin to refine the stress that used to define you. The masterpiece that is now your life didn't happen all at once but has unfolded moment by moment—so let's give those moments the attention they deserve.

MEDITATION MEAL #1
Breathe

⌒∽

What is it and why is my seventeen-year-old doing it?

I remember the day I walked into my seventeen-year-old son's room to awkwardly tell him I was writing a book on meditation. This wavy-haired starter for the high school football team started scrolling through his phone.

I took two unphased steps backward before hearing his "Wait, Mom!" What he proceeded to show me on his phone changed my view of meditation. The meditation app he was already using to calm and refocus was a surprise to me; but then again, his generation was born into a sea of distraction, and it's no surprise they would eventually reach a breaking point and find a way of calming the chaos. My generation can at least remember what it was like before the stressors we have today as we move from Mayberry to mayhem in just half a lifetime. The good news is that "meditation" is now a household word, heard in Hollywood interviews and used by big, burly farmer-types. It's no longer a taboo topic, but for beginners, it is important to understand what meditation is.

Meditation trains the brain the way your fitness program trains your body. You see value in treating your physical body well, but most of us do not know how to treat our brain well by tapping into the limitless supply of inner peace that exists in all of us. The controlled and slowed breathing of morning meditation brings us closer to our natural, peaceful state—a place of existence that is crucial for brain-wellness. If you haven't seen that peaceful state in a while, it's because it is hiding beneath the strong forces of frustrations, obligations, and anxiety that have built up in us over time. The key to finding that place of peace beneath the crusty chaos is in your breath. Training the brain starts with breathing in, holding the breath, and slowly breathing out.

Meditation brings clarity to our thoughts. As busy humans with active brains that turn on the moment our feet hit the floor each day, thoughts can get in the way of morning meditation. Whereas other publications describe meditation as pushing your thoughts away and creating an empty space, I experience meditation as shining a light of clarity upon existing thoughts. This approach gives our thoughts new perspective and new life, much like a cloudy day when the fog begins to fade and a ray of sunlight shines through. We all love that moment after endless days of winter or rain when the warm sunshine hits our face for the first time. Our brain spends much of its time in a fog of completing tasks and going through routines, but like glorious sunshine, meditation breaks through the fog every morning. In these moments of focused, slow breathing, a bright light shines on the many thoughts in our brain, making them clear and fresh.

One of my businesses demands constant creativity in order to grow. Before discovering meditation, my creative moments happened on vacation only. I found it strange that the creative juices flowed nonstop while on a break from work. It was great to return to work with lots of fresh ideas, but I could not help but wonder what was stopping the flow at work. After incorporating meditation into my daily routine, everything changed. The moment I reach a place of peace each morning where my thoughts are illuminated, the creativity starts to overflow. I now have so many "Ah-ha" moments that I have to keep a notebook nearby during meditation. The more you meditate, the clearer the thoughts become. Quickly you will discover that receiving a fresh approach to existing thoughts makes your living room feel like you have a room with a view.

Meditation creates a connection. The great thing about meditation is that it transcends belief systems and any preconceived notions of spirituality. It is natural to feel a connection during meditation, especially when you need help, physical healing, or personal peace. Most people initially attempt to meditate simply to alleviate anxiety, but as you master the art of meditation, you discover connections as a surprising and welcome side effect. Who or what you connect with depends on you. Whether connecting with God, a loved one who has passed, a guardian angel, or the universe in general, the connection is personal and belongs to you.

During the 1980s, my best friend and I were in high school. She begged me to enter the annual talent show with her and, although neither of us had any real talent to speak of, we spent hours practicing a routine, stopping only to push play on her cassette player over and over again. Seven years later, she passed away. Although I cannot help but think of her on occasion, it was not until I began to meditate that a connected memory of our talent show escapades came to mind one morning. A few hours later, I jumped in a cab to head to an appointment, and wouldn't you know it? That 80s hit that we played over and over in practice was playing as I got into the car. I smiled as I connected with my dear friend. Coincidence? Maybe, but it's my moment, and you will have plenty of undisputed ones of your own.

I was twenty-five when my friend died, and I had never even been to a funeral. Still full of sadness and questions, I never expected another, even more painful tragedy to happen within a month's time. When my dad passed away unexpectedly, I transitioned from sadness to anger. Why would God take such a good one? How would I be able to live without this man who supported us, made us laugh daily, and set a standard of integrity for my brothers and sister and myself? He was the cornerstone of our family. He was snatched away far too soon and would not be present to walk me down the aisle or meet his grandchildren. I spent too much time being angry with God.

Years passed before I allowed myself to notice the influence my dad was having on our lives even after his death. It was as if he was patiently waiting for me to make a connection (a strange concept for this preppy Presbyterian who had grown up talking to God, not dead people.) Meditation opened a positive connection for me that allowed me to ask for help from the many masters who have passed away. Death will always be painful for the living, but making a connection through meditation softens the blow. The universe has your back!

Can just six minutes really change my morning?

Yes! Meditation Meal #1 creates a clear focus for your day. The choices you make upon waking not only set the tone for your day but allow you to control your day instead of your day controlling you. Sure, we all oversleep on occasion and have to rush into work mode, but those are the days that start off on the wrong foot and need to be avoided. Getting up twenty minutes earlier can move mountains in terms of your attitude about your day. The world is loud and distracting, creating a need for you to decompress. A quick, easy morning meditation gives you the upper hand on your day.

With today's mental to-do list unfolding as you slam the alarm clock, it is tempting to skip the morning meditation and rush into action. Deadlines, anticipation of duties, and things forgotten from yesterday trick us into thinking that a few extra minutes in the morning is simply not feasible. Actually, the opposite is true. For just a minimum of six minutes, meditation can ease the stress of the morning in a way that will surprise you. Believe me, you will still meet your deadline—but this time without overhauling your digestive system.

Meditation Meal #1 is an instrument for energy. You would think that slow breathing in the early morning hours would zap your energy, counteract your coffee, and send you snoring again. Instead, by calming the mind, a higher quality energy emerges, giving you that new and clear perspective on your day. Think about the energy you have when you hear you closed a deal or got offered a new, exciting opportunity. This type of energy propels you to jump into action. Now picture your boss yelling at you for forgetting an important task and how you fly into action to complete it with a different type of energy. Meditation brings out the good kind of energy, the one that comes from a space within and sends you into your day with true joy.

A morning meditation a day keeps the doctor away. When I asked my seventeen-year-old why he was using a meditation app on his phone, he responded with all things physical. My son and I both suffered from migraine headaches for years. From the time he was very young, he began a pattern of missing school a couple of days each month due to migraines, and outside forces never solved the problem. Stress and anxiety have a sneaky way of affecting our body, and for my son, the meditation app worked wonders. It set him free from the pain of weekly headaches. I'm not here to try and explain the well-documented mind-body connection, but experience is everything. If meditation makes you feel better, then it is worth the few minutes you spend each day. The more connected you are with yourself through meditation, the more likely you are to feel healthy and happy.

Six Meditation Meals a Day began as a personal journey for me, and because it completely changed my medical chart, I am sharing what worked for me in the hope that someone else can also benefit from fewer doctor visits and feeling great regardless of the amount of stress in our day.

In 2008, I took a chance in life: I left a stable job with benefits and a retirement fund. Starting a business from scratch is scary, and the type of stress that emerges is brutal compared to the stable kind of stress. As a single mom with two kids to support, it was truly up to me to make this leap of faith and not fall flat in front of my family, friends, and two young boys. Even when success finally arrives, the stress remains as a hovering reminder not to get too comfortable. Stress showed itself in the form of migraines, nightmares, and a very complicated digestive system. Medications and other outside remedies proved to be ineffective, and the medical mysteries continued. Doctor visit after doctor visit revealed no concrete answers and only pulled me away from work, which made the stress worse since I was behind and had to work overtime to catch up.

I felt like I was headed down a road to a heart attack. When you are self employed, it is easy to take on more when opportunities arise because you think you can handle it, but more success means more stress. You welcome the success but never anticipate the stress that tags along with it. I knew I needed to do something to stop the cycle of stress, and I didn't like the person I was when agitated and angry with my family, employees, and even strangers. Knowing that there is something more out there and desperately needing a solution led me to search for an answer that was there all along.

I am happy to say that, solely because of pausing daily to complete six small meditation meals a day, I have healed all the areas causing me pain and frustration. No more migraines, no more waking in the middle of the night in a panic, and no more probing doctors. No more thousands spent on medical bills and no more unpredictability about where the stress-related illnesses will show up next. There is great joy in feeling healthy, and it is meditation that has brought me to this happy place. Stress will continue to be present in our lives and we may never be able to fully eliminate stress, but through meditation, there is a drastic change to the way we view the stress and the people and factors causing it. *Six Small Meditation Meals a Day* allows you to weigh the degree of stress you feel and puts you in a healthy place of control as you manage your day in a meditative way!

Just do it and don't forget to breathe

If you experience stress throughout your day, you owe it to yourself to try meditation. Keep in mind that the active brain has a harder time at first with adjusting to meditation, but it needs meditation the most. The best way to start is to vow to try with no expectation. Create a judgment-free zone in terms of your thoughts, trust the process, and give yourself a little slack. Just as food is used to accomplish six small meals during the day, so is the breath utilized to master six small meditations throughout the day.

Beginners need nothing more than to breathe in, hold for six or seven seconds, and breathe out. I find it helpful to envision a stream of bright, golden light filling my body as I breathe in. As I breathe out, I picture a gray stream containing all the negative junk and stress leaving my body. Focus on the change you want in your life, and in just six minutes each morning, you will transform yourself from the inside out.

Here's the Meat of MM#1: Six Minutes

Find a comfortable place in the early morning hours. With your eyes closed and back straight, begin to breathe in and hold for seven seconds. As you breathe in, imagine drawing in a bright yellow light that fills your body. Then, imagine breathing out a gray, cloudy stream that symbolizes whatever no longer serves you any positive purpose. Repeat.

MEDITATION MEAL #2
Immunity

⌒

TJ's morning meditation was successful. He took a quick drive through Java Jeff's and was still ahead of schedule. Downtown traffic was less busy than usual in his booming town, and his favorite song hit the waves as he turned into the bank's corporate lot. He didn't even care that new intern parking was the farthest away—it was already a great day.

It was his second week of a prestigious paid internship, and this rising junior was already being solicited by several big banks. Stress was fresh for this young go-getter still getting care packages from mom, but his 8 a.m. smile was greeted with a look of concern from his project manager. The numbers he had worked on for way too many hours yesterday were off by a fraction of a percentage, resulting in a mistake that could affect thousands of dollars.

"Plan to stay well into the evening today," his manager declared.

When TJ, a former employee, told me about the first fifteen minutes of his day, I knew he needed a tool to protect himself just as much as those of us who had already hardened to the crusty layers of stress.

Meditation Meal #2—*Immunity* is designed to ground and protect you from the bombardment of the start of the workday. Even just three minutes to ground yourself before you walk into that classroom or boardroom or tackle a stack of papers a mile high can create an immunity to stress mid-morning and diffuse the dense fog that typically creeps in between MM#1 and MM#2. That type of fog prevents you from seeing the direction of your goals clearly and hinders the creative ideas that will grow your business or improve your work environment. With an immunity meditation, you focus on this morning only and allow future worries to dissipate. That which used to throw you off your game is no longer a challenge. Eyes open, eyes closed, walking into work, or pausing in a bathroom stall—a quick two- or three-minute meditation is the metaphorical equivalent of putting on a suit of armor.

As you bring back your breath around 9:30 a.m. each day, you become fully present in this moment. For me, 9:30 a.m. means going from calm to chaos in just a matter of minutes, and the quick mini-meditation makes all the difference in how I respond and handle the stress. Here are three things I do as part of an immunity meditation:

Antidote for adrenaline

We high-octane humans don't really need caffeine, do we? Yet a warm cup of our favorite fluid gives us something to look forward to when the alarm clock sounds. I just plain do not want to give it up. Therefore, part of my MM#2 is to make sure I haven't gone too far. A quick assessment of our calm-o-meter will help gauge how prepared we are for unexpected morning stress, which can be made worse when we are overdosing on adrenaline.

Check your pulse, grab a bottle of water, and sneak in a mini-meditation that focuses on calming your entire body. Begin to feel your body relax from head to toe. Even just thirty seconds of controlled breathing before the winds of the workplace move in allow you to diffuse the adrenaline-based reactions. During this moment of focus, repeat to yourself, "*Respond instead of react.*"

This morning, you are making the conscious effort to respond and not react. Remind yourself that most of your reactions are based on your past experiences, good or bad. See your reaction for what it is and be open to understanding the reaction of others as they have had their own past experiences that influence the way they react to you. Respond from where you are now, not where you used to be.

Strap on your blinders

Just like the leather flaps on a horse-halter keep it from seeing too much at a time, we need to train the brain to focus on this morning only. When you are high energy and super motivated, this is not an easy task. You see into next week, next year, and today's mental to-do list just grew to three pages. The highly motivated are naturally attracted to an array of opportunities and so many enticing options. It is hard to say no when we are confident in our ability to handle more. But doing so can send our energy in so many directions that we become weakened overall, unknowingly setting ourselves up for a mental overload. Strapping on blinders mid-morning focuses our attention on one thing at a time and pulls our head out of next week. With all your energy being poured into the work of this morning only, the tasks of today receive a creative spotlight instead of a dim flicker formerly brought on by our diffused energy.

As the workday begins, stress can often be at the day's highest level due to over-scheduling. Whereas a tainted timeline creates frustration, a simple change in mindset can allow you to proceed calmly toward the success you already know how to create. You are the person to accomplish it all but MM#2 protects the positive progress you have made toward your goals while keeping you harnessed to the tasks of today. With blinders on, make a conscious choice to be fully aware and present in the tasks and conversations of this morning. When you raise your awareness, you create a connection to those around you, allowing you to see what truly matters in this part of your day.

Blinders at MM#2 also appease tomorrow's financial woes as you calmly remind yourself that you have made it this far and things will continue to increase in the future. Mentally blinding yourself from the stressors of tomorrow or even later today allows you to set correct intentions for morning appointments and activities. You can give your people the attention and attitude they deserve and expect from the true you.

Code switching

Of the three quick exercises I do as part of MM#2, this one is most important. The concept of Code Switching, or easing from one language to another, is common among the bilingual. A bank teller speaks one way at work with her customers and slips seamlessly into the language of her home and close friends after work is over. An Alabama college student studying in NYC can assimilate quickly on his return to southern culture. On a more basic level, a call from a client sounds different than a call from your best bud. I use the same concept of code switching to address the stress.

As a busy human, you are more likely to float around in ego mode. In fact, we thrive in ego mode. We direct, lead, hire and fire, serve on more than one committee, and accomplish more in one day than most people. You are a confident person who seizes opportunities and knows how to create the life you desire.

The most powerful immunity that protects the positive progress toward your goals, however, happens when you turn inward to your true self—your soul mode. By stepping *outside* the ego to get *inside* to the soul, the stress of mid-morning is replaced with the listening ear to intuition, one of your greatest assets. Most people do not know that it is even possible to exist in any other state, and yet we have the ability and choice to feel peaceful at any time, not just after work or once the kids have gone to bed.

I mentally flip a switch from ego to soul every morning around 9:30 a.m.

Using your "soul sense" will cause you to calmly approach the tasks of today.

Ego approaches the chaos with anger and frustration and is easily offended by others' opinions. Soul is neither offended nor reacts hastily to this morning's surprises. Soul knows you are exactly where you are meant to be this morning and that there is nothing coming your way today that you cannot handle. Soul is flexible, whereas the ego is rigid and frustrated by unexpected change.

A conscious soul switch allows you to increase awareness in your present moments of the morning, leading employees or coworkers to view you as fully connected instead of distracted and consumed by obligations.

The key is in the slip from one mode to another. As you perfect the switch, soul will begin to emerge at all the right times, allowing you to rise above the chaos and thus creating efficiency in your morning. Believe me, your employees, co-workers, spouse, etc. will reap the awesome side effects!

Many of the great healers, spiritual advisors, and inspiring authors have been able to remove themselves from day-to-day chaos and create an ego-less environment that helps them thrive. For some of us, that's not an option, so learning how to code switch from ego to soul is a must-have skill for every busy person. Unlike publications that urge throwing out the ego completely, I believe we need an element of ego. That part of us that makes things happen and explains why they pay us the big bucks is important.

As you master the art of the switch from ego to soul, you will eventually slip seamlessly from one mode to another. To be a true master of the switch is to know when to be in soul mode, your most noble mode. For it is in soul mode where your true self exists, the one that really matters. With a little practice, you will discover that even in ego mode, you become less irritable, less arrogant, and much less quick to anger.

MM#2—*Immunity* is about protecting yourself from stress mid-morning and being aware of the people and duties needing your full attention. It is about remembering that your reactions are based on past experiences and approaching future reactions with a responsive calm. Immunity is slipping seamlessly from ego to soul at just the right moment and finding your center of peace during any storm.

Mastering the immunity meditation mid-morning strengthens your ability to handle the unexpected and the undesired. Your thoughts are now clear, making all responses to problems sound and efficient. When you are no longer distracted by the afternoon or tomorrow, your focus becomes fine-tuned and your creative juices begin to overflow. Remember all the great ideas you came up with while staring into the vastness of the ocean or the peace you felt watching bison roam the fields below a mighty mountain backdrop? These same innovations flow freely in the workplace when you allow just a few minutes for an immunity meditation to become part of your mid-morning routine. The time and effort you have invested in your work deserves to be protected.

Here's the Intel on MM#2: Three Minutes
Slip into a bathroom stall and bring back the breath. Short and simple will make a big difference. As your breath comes in, allow a soft green light to fill your heart area and calm your reactions. Mentally strap on your blinders. Who needs your attention this morning? Bring awareness to this mid-morning routine and turn the switch from ego to soul.

MEDITATION MEAL #3
Inspire

⁓

nspiration is the catalyst for pushing us forward in life, and although it comes in many forms and from many places, we all have a need to be inspired. Our elders inspire us to choose integrity over success. A friend who has survived insurmountable events inspires us to be grateful. A song can inspire us to dance with our spouse, and a good book inspires us to think differently. A person in need may inspire us to be more giving; a successful colleague will inspire us to work harder.

From the Latin *inspiritus,* our word "inspire" means "the drawing of air into the breath." You perfected this technique in the morning meditation (MM#1— *Breathe*), which focused on clarity of thoughts and connecting with yourself or others through breath. MM#2—*Immunity* helped draw the air into your lungs to guard and prepare you for workday stress. MM#3— *Inspire* brings back the breath once again, this time with a focus on inspiration. Typically performed during a midday hour, a sweet Inspire notification reminds you to pause and take ten minutes to be inspired.

MM#3 incorporates a mental break alongside a physical lunch break usually viewed as insignificant in a busy day, a quick bite to eat while in a client meeting, running errands across town, or catching up on paperwork. MM#3 reminds you to keep inspiration alive by turning your humdrum ham and cheese into magical moments of inspiration! Having a secured time each day to allow yourself to be inspired takes wasted and ordinary midday moments to an extraordinary level that instantly calms the stress.

Unlike the morning meditation (MM#1), which is consistent in its design and methods, MM#3 can take on a new direction every day and is dependent upon circumstances and schedules. You may find yourself in unexpected places at the midday hour when your notification sounds—dealing with an unexpected delivery truck, a long-distance phone call, or an overdue oil change. When inspiration is your focus, the circumstances may vary, but your mission to seek a better you prevails. Let the inspiration begin!

Put the oxygen mask on yourself first
MM#3 begins with taking care of your own inspiration. We are creative by nature, but busy schedules can hinder our ability to be inspired, and yet daily creative

time is key to moving forward both professionally and personally. We spend so much time daily in the fog of doing tasks and getting our day done that we leave little room for the type of thinking that really matters.

A teacher who takes time to inspire herself turns textbook boredom into a classroom of engaged learners who look forward to her class each day. A business owner who replaces task time with creative time will rise above his competitors who remain stationary on the carousel of their career. A busy mom who takes time to inspire herself while folding laundry will give her kids an inspiration they will remember long after they outgrow their clothes.

MM#3 pulls you off the treadmill of life and gives you a gift of daily time focused solely on the type of inspiration that propels you to a better place in life. What this personal time looks like depends on you but always begins with bringing back the breath and then choosing your moment of enrichment.

In the early 90s, I can remember laughing at the antics of comedian Steve Martin, so when an email came across my inbox almost thirty years later with his face, I took notice. He was hosting a Master Class. Stand-up comedy was never my goal, but I was intrigued by the chance to have intimate online video time with the great Steve Martin. Laughter is healing for stress, and his course in comedy became my ten-minute inspiration each day for several weeks at 12:30 p.m.—and yes, my one-liners at the water cooler were getting noticed.

Find what speaks to you. Engaging with a creative think-tank focused on a new business idea leads to time spent in an invaluable way, as is reading several pages in a new book, listening to a TED Talk, or simply researching a topic of interest. The inspiration is limitless. Whether your ten minutes each day is spent inspiring yourself professionally or personally, the goal of this meditation is to use creative inspiration to calm the stress, preparing you for a productive afternoon. Let your 12:30 p.m. notification remind you to guard this time each day before stepping back on your treadmill. Inspiration is the destination for this meditation, but the direction you take to get there is up to you.

Inspiring others

Only once you have inspired yourself will you be able to inspire others. This is a selfless act often given with no knowledge of its effects. When you take a minute to think of all the people and places that have inspired you along the way, the names may have faded but the effect on your life remains. The inspiration even total strangers can provide can be powerful enough to significantly impact a person's life.

My parents were in denial, and I was too young to recognize the effects that drugs were having on my older brother who drove me to school each day. It was the mid-70's and his speeding Ford and blaring 8-track player hindered any bond between the two of us. A few years later, I ended up with that old Maverick and worn out tape player while he was hours away at college where we knew even less about the struggles he faced.

Thanks to the inspiration of others and the time they took to notice and encourage him without reward, my brother went on to be one of the greatest men I know, pastoring a large non-denominational church where he is an inspiration to thousands of people every day.

Inspiring others is not planned ahead and is as simple as interacting with people in a way that raises their level of good energy by affirming them, complimenting them, and showing respect for who they are. Every person in your life and every person you encounter midday needs to hear the equivalent of, "Great job!" Whether complimenting a new outfit, an initiative taken on the job, or noticing a kind gesture by a coworker, you have the power to inspire others. There is not a person alive who doesn't respond to praise. Even the guy who "has it all" goes shoulders up when someone compliments his perfectly grilled grouper.

Inspiring others is not about approaching random strangers or imparting all your worldly wisdom in one breakroom monologue. A sentence here or a compliment there creates a connection with your coworker, employee, or cashier at the coffee shop. Your midday notification instantly acts as a reminder to become self-aware and that when you are not inspiring yourself, you can seek to inspire someone else. You might be just what another person needed in this moment on his or her journey, and even if you never know the effect you are having, trust that the universe is using you for good.

Here's the Fuel for MM#3:
Inspire for Ten Minutes

It's lunchtime, and instead of simply cramming in a chicken salad, bring back the breath and breathe in the flame of inspiration, hold for seven seconds, and let out the foggy matter of "routine brain." It's up to you to inspire yourself. Choose your focus today and spend a few moments creatively—learning, reading, or listening while eating your lunch.

Perhaps it's 12:30 p.m. and you are at a crowded lunch counter. As you wash your hands in the restroom, bring back the breath and hold. Release all the frustration that has built up since 9:30 a.m. Repeat these steps. Return to your seat aware of the journey of those around you and see their souls, not their faces. Let your heart guide you to inspire another person today.

MEDITATION MEAL #4
Big Picture

❧

I t is one hour before closing time and you are reminding yourself once more not to buy that brand of printer ever again. You feel overwhelmed and there is still too much to do before the end of the day. It's time to bring back the breath once again for this three-minute meditation around 4 p.m. daily. Can the frustration you feel attach itself to an event from earlier today? Does the tension in your neck have a name? I incorporate two quick techniques as part of MM#4. The first is a quick body scan that allows you to assess the stress that has been building since the morning and search for the lessons amidst the chaos. The second takes you high above your life where a new perspective emerges.

See struggles as lessons

In order to address the stress using MM#4, we must change the way we view the stress in our lives. I believe life is school for the soul, which means struggles are opportunities to learn and grow. Just simply seeing stressful situations as part of the universe's attempt to move and stretch your understanding drastically changes the way you see the situation. What used to cause anger and high blood pressure now causes you to step back and see something else happening altogether.

For instance, when I was writing this section of the book, my worst nightmare came true. The universe has our backs, but apparently the Big U also has a sense of humor. One of my businesses involves hosting events for large groups, and I have often told the staff about my horrible dream of a group showing up that was not on our schedule and taking us by complete surprise.

Just imagine one hundred people coming to your backyard for a private party, unannounced, with you completely unaware. Yep, it happened—and that is when you pull out the big guns of MM#4. Using the *Big Picture* method allowed me to see this very stressful situation as a soul lesson in responding with a calm solution instead of reacting with panic and accusation. You, too, will face many struggles in this school of life. In fact, once you pass a test, more tests will come. As life presents you with new challenges, your big-picture view of stress will allow you to see the difficult situations as opportunities to grow.

We have all been given different life lessons, and no one is exempt from these struggles—even whom those we view as having an easy life. We are all at different points in our journey, and it is important not to judge the journey of another. What may be difficult for you to handle may be easily accepted by your coworker. Those things that make you question, "Why is this happening to me?" are things you can handle, and they are the very things leading to a greater version of you.

Even those who are truly in tune with the universe encounter frustrations and disappointments. The difference is, they have a better understanding of the fact that despite the chaos and stress, all things in their lives are divinely where they are supposed to be. When struggles become lessons, the way you react to people and events is transformed. Instead of popping blood vessels, your response is calm and mindful of another perspective. It is helpful to weigh the degree of stress you feel and compare it to events on the nightly news. Updating your view of your own stress can drastically change the way you view your struggle. Suddenly, the situations and people causing you stress seem to ease away.

This is when deeper change begins to occur. Not only will the people in your life notice that your anger has dissipated, but your doctor will begin to miss you. One of the greatest benefits of mini-meditation meals for me personally has been the huge transformation in my medical journey. I am certain that my ability to change the way I view the mounting stress in my life has led to complete healing of migraines, anxiety-induced nightmares, and a complicated digestive system. I still experience an overwhelming amount of stress on a regular basis, but changing the way I view the stress as part of MM#4 has truly set me free.

Pelican perspective

In addition to finding the lessons in the stressors of the morning, I utilize a quick technique I call the Pelican Perspective. We tend to see only our day, our week, or this past year. In addition, our human bodies limit us from seeing a bigger picture for our lives. A pelican perspective skyrockets our spirit and mind high above our lives where a new perspective emerges, reminding us of how insignificant our little frustrations from earlier today really are. See yourself and the situations causing the stress. Look to the right and then left and see all the many people around you going through their situations and struggles. As you float above your life, this new aerial attitude causes the anger and aggravations to instantly disappear.

Several years ago, my dream property went up for sale. I just knew I was meant to get this piece of property and was confident the universe would somehow make it happen. You can imagine my surprise when I found out that within days of being listed, it was already under contract. Someone else would get this property, and I was left upset and feeling abandoned (I may have even stomped a little). I had been so certain about my vision for this property that I was left confused about the universe's plan and why it was not working out in my favor.

Flash forward four years later and the same property went up for sale again! This time, I was not only in a much better place financially but now had an entirely fresh vision for this property, one that had not existed in my mind four years earlier. In fact, I can see clearly now that if that property had been mine the first time around, I would have made a major business mistake that could have cost me thousands. I am grateful to the Big U for overriding my limited view and guiding me through what I could not see in that moment. I didn't have a pelican perspective back then, but having one would have helped me to avoid the anger, tears, and a little foot stomping. You are small and the universe is big. If your plan is overturned, it wasn't the right plan!

MM#4—*Big Picture* means changing the way you view stress, opening yourself up to new perspectives, and seeing life from a much bigger vantage point, and this all can be done in just three minutes or less. It will not make the stress go away nor will it guarantee you leave work on time, but it will replace anger with trust, enabling you to know you are exactly where you need to be in life. Your personal journey will continue to have difficulties and disappointments. But with a pelican perspective and a new understanding of what your struggles are trying to teach you, the stress is replaced with a connected understanding of a bigger plan.

We can never completely prepare ourselves for the unexpected disappointments, the losses, and the aggravations, but we can plan ahead for how we will react. Having a new perspective toward our stress and a view from above is the key to this afternoon meditation. Find peace in knowing that no matter how bad or confusing the situation appears to you, things are, in fact, in perfect order.

Here's the Skinny on Big Picture Meditation: Three Minutes

Breathe in, hold for six to seven seconds, and release. As you calm your body, quickly assess today's struggles and search for what the universe is trying to teach you during this struggle. What did you learn from the Big U today? Fly high above your body and see how small your problem really is amid a much bigger picture. Find peace in knowing you are exactly where you need to be.

MEDITATION MEAL #5
Purposeful Indulgence
(with Gratitude)

MM#5 focuses on taking time to reward yourself after a typical day where demands are extreme and the body has been pushed beyond a healthy level. We busy humans accept the stress but rarely schedule time to decompress. As you scroll through your calendar for today, I'm guessing you will find obligations and appointments lined up throughout today—but not one of them has you looking out for yourself. MM#5 is a 7 p.m. meditation designed to be a guilt-free span of indulgence with an emphasis on gratitude. Allowing your body to smile after the stress you encounter is a mighty goal for some high-octane humans, but when paired with the power of gratitude, this break becomes one of the highlights of your day.

The more stressful the day, the earlier in the day we should plan for MM#5. This allows us to look forward to something that makes us happy near the end of the workday. This meditation and focus point will help restore balance and, when paired with humility and gratitude, it gives you the freedom to make yourself happy. Three hours have passed since your last mini-meditation, but the obligations of home and work have crept back in, bringing tension along as its guest. The fact that you are aware of stress and do not like it in your life is a healthy sign that you are paying attention to the signals your body is giving you.

By 7 p.m., it is time to bring back the breath once again and focus on a meditation that makes you smile each time you hear the sweet notification for MM#5. Making time for your own needs soothes the physical body and feeds your spirit.

Make self-care a priority

Most of us do not make a conscious effort to guard time daily for ourselves, but neglecting the self will eventually catch up with us. Making MM#5 a priority each day and indulging in pre-planned self-care will bring out the happy and send the stress flying. Eventually you will not even notice your evening habit reminder because you will be one step ahead of the notification, fully engaged in what personally brings you enjoyment each day.

Even on the easy days or the ones we think are stress-free, self-care needs to be a routine. Exercise after work, an occasional massage, or time spent decluttering your happy place are all ways to take care of you and you alone. Sure, it seems crazy that we have to use a notification to remind ourselves to make self-care a daily priority, but more success brings more stress. We welcome the success but rarely notice the effects of stress until it's too late. Begin today to give back to yourself by reacting to your 7 p.m. notification and make MM#5 mandatory each day.

Reconnect with your passions

One of the best ways to indulge yourself after a stressful day is to reconnect with something you love to do, something that is truly a part of who you are. MM#5 sets a daily reminder to bring back the breath with a smile as you focus on what activities will allow your full engagement and reconnect you with your personal passions.

What activities seriously make you smile? List them in your mind and quickly cross out the ones that involve flying across the country to satisfy (save that list for later). Enjoy a beverage on your back porch, read five pages in the book you started on vacation and never finished, or allow that guitar sitting in the corner to take you back to a summer night on the lake. Exercise and animals are both known to reduce stress, and the dog always needs more (not less) walking. Engaging in something after work that makes you happy moves mountains in the land of stress.

It helps to think back to when you were a kid. When the fun was happening, you were fully engaged, not analyzing your actions like we do as adults. Pure fun as a kid didn't come in the manufactured form of bright lights and big events. It was found in the endless laughter of our own backyards. Like the kid waiting for the sprinkler to turn over and over, entertained for hours without a care, allow yourself to engage in your own passion where there is no room for worry in your thoughts. Indulging in something you are passionate about once a day does not mean you have to act like a kid, but as you find yourself fully present in your passion, you might actually catch yourself screaming, "Do it again!"

Gratitude

If life has put you in a fortunate position to engage in much needed self-care or indulge in childlike passions, then *gratitude* must be your companion. I remember when the word "gratitude" was a word of intention a few years ago and was popping up on signs, pillows, and bracelets. For many people like me, it was a positive spark that created awareness of how gratitude was being manifested in my life. Gratitude allows the indulgence to never be taken for granted. When gratitude is paired with indulgence, you are given the freedom to make yourself happy. Gratitude is the key factor that takes your indulgence from guilty pleasure to a moment of self-care each evening.

Anticipation softens the blow

Purposely planning a daily indulgence creates a secured happy time that you will look forward to from the moment your day begins. The more stressful the day, the earlier and more specific the indulgence can be intentionally planned for after work. Having something to look forward to softens the stress throughout the day. Creating a positive anticipation each day makes the unexpected blows or aggravating appointments a little less painful.

Kids are masters at positive anticipation. They blindly bounce through their days entirely engrossed in waiting for the next exciting thing—the next holiday, birthday, or fun event. I can't get my kids to work on their social studies project the week before it's due, but they have no trouble handing me a double-spaced, prioritized Christmas list complete with links for online purchases. Use MM#5 as a tool to be kind to yourself daily, engage in activities that stir up passion, and be grateful.

> **Here's the Icing on MM#5: Fifteen Minutes**
> Breathe in, hold for seven seconds, and breathe out, releasing all the tension in the neck and shoulders. As you breathe in again, choose a way to indulge yourself in self-care today. Feel the gratitude and let it calm your entirely thankful body. Spend at least fifteen minutes reconnecting with your passion or doing something for yourself that makes you smile.

MEDITATION MEAL #6
Clearing

∾

H ome is a place we look forward to after a long day's work. It is a safe haven from the people and events that have caused us frustration, and as we pass through the threshold of our homes, we assume all is well and that we have arrived at a place guaranteed to be relaxing and free of stress. A cold beer on a TV tray fools us into thinking the stress is really gone.

What we are not able to see is the mental build-up that has followed us home from work. Those thick layers that have been accumulating all day on our outer bodies make it hard to ease the mind late in the day, and without clearing this invisible crust, a sleepless night is sure to follow.

MM#6—*Clearing* is an evening meditation that will allow you to discover how to quiet the mind to get to your soul at the end of a long day. This quick but intentional break in our evening pattern not only sends you into a more peaceful rest, it allows today to have a finite end and tomorrow to have a fresh perspective. Unlike the morning meditations which are full of anticipation and energy for a new day of possibilities, the evening often finds us reeling from the disappointments, frustrations, and unrecognized anxiety that have formed a crust on the creative person we were just hours ago. If you are a highly sensitive person, the hidden deposits of mental anguish are even worse.

When we have a *good* day, we have no problem posting and proclaiming to our friends and family all that is going well, but with a *bad* day, all the energy is turned inward, piled upon ourselves. Good days make us feel like we are on the right course and all that is happening is meant to be, but bad days leave us feeling abandoned by the universe. The good news is that despite the struggles and very rotten days, daily lessons will continue to abound, moving you to a better place in life. In fact, it is on those very worst days when the universe not only has your back but is pulling you out of a stagnant place. MM#6 helps you to trade those feelings of abandonment with an understanding that struggles will make you stronger and create new learning.

MM#6—*Clearing* is the key to removing the coating at the end of the day, and for just a few meditative minutes, a quick evaluation of your day with the purpose of clearing the junky build-up can prepare you for a great tomorrow. Whether it happens while relaxing in your bed or in the brief moments in your home office as you unplug for the night, these few minutes of clearing can drastically change your quality of sleep.

Stress is unpredictable and rarely arrives in equal amounts. Each day, the demands for clearing can vary. I break down MM#6 into two levels: Heavy Clearing and Light Clearing. Paying attention to the signals your body is giving you and turning an inward ear to intuition will give you clarity as to the type of clearing you need. There is ease on the days of light clearing, but when you are equipped to handle the heavy clearing needed on the really aggravating days, the stress no longer creeps into your sleep; with a little practice, you will be prepared to take on even the worst of days.

Heavy clearing

Some days are definitely worse than others. When you are in a position to make things go a certain way at work or at home, clearing can be a challenge. When our plan is not going as expected, we tend to force the plan, which makes letting go during MM#6 more difficult. A heavy clearing is crucial for those in control of employees, programs, or production as well as for the meal-skipper and the multitasker. On the days where there is frustration, aggravation, and anger, a heavy clearing is a must, and we can no longer assume that we are leaving everything that bothers us behind as we enter our homes. The high-hope energy of the morning has faded by the end of the day, and MM#6 replaces your depleted energy, with the restoring power of life's energy sending you into a peaceful and worry-free sleep! I utilize three techniques as part of a heavy clearing.

No Vacancy

Sherry started as a cashier at a large retail store thirty miles outside of Charlotte. She was efficient and focused—and management took notice, moving her into an assistant position within her first year. By the time I met Sherry, she was head of customer service, and many people would say she had achieved much in just a few short years. But when I sat next to her at a business luncheon, she struck a chord with me when she mentioned that she often daydreams about her days as a cashier.

The stress that comes with success can be overwhelming, but imagining trading a higher salary for stress relief seemed like an unnecessary thought process. I knew Sherry needed to incorporate a No Vacancy attitude as part of her nightly clearing. This mental tool is especially crucial for all the Sherrys of the world.

Later, as you lay on your pillow to quiet your soul, don't be afraid to call out the causes of your stress by name.Simply identifying the reasons for your frustrations is the first step to keeping these people and situations from renting space in your head. Picture yourself holding a "No Vacancy" sign, and every challenging relationship and all the anger attached to people is pushed away as they are not allowed to enter your space. As you bring back the breath in MM#6, they may try to sneak past the front desk, but they are pushed away as you exhale. It is important to create a space of clearing that allows you to be truly free of the people and events that cause you pain. Mentally mount your No Vacancy sign over your headboard and keep pushing the squatters off your bed as you drift off to sleep.

Five-Year Flashback
A second technique I use as part of an evening clearing meditation is a tool that reminds you how far you have come. Regularly remembering the struggles of several years ago can help ease the blows of today's hardship. As you breathe in, flashback to five years ago and observe your life as an outsider. Retrospection is a healing tool, for what you could not see then is seen clearly now.

Notice how the universe had your back then and how much you have learned from the things you thought were simply struggles. Focus on the growth of the past five years as a way of reminding yourself that you are *exactly* where you are supposed to be in this moment and then bask in the tranquility of your transformation. If you want to really blow your mind, turn back to ten years!

You are a person who is moving forward, but when you are focused on the aggravations of today, that progress is slowed by the fog of frustration. The stress that comes with success clouds your brain in the late evening, but you have several tools to push the fog away. Remembering how far you've come as you breathe is a great place to start.

Find Three to Set You Free

Two hurricanes and a relentless amount of rain in the fall of 2018 had weathermen in awe of record-breaking levels of rising waters not seen in my lifetime. This became a recipe for fear for businesses and farmers across the US who had never before needed to trust in a sunny tomorrow. I had a personal loss of thousands but seeing the water-soaked fields and faces of the farmers in the Carolinas was humbling. As the waters continued to rise so did the fear of finances and any meditation became distracted and difficult. It is not easy to trust that the future is taken care of when you are wrapped in a blanket of disbelief. In extreme times of struggle when it seems there is little light giving you hope, I utilize a third strategy in a Heavy Clearing— *Find Three to Set You Free*.

This simple exercise allows you to find perspective in the midst of fear and frustration when stress is at its worst and the previous two strategies in a heavy clearing are not enough. It is natural to base our success on the tangible, but really bad days call for identifying the intangible: the things you have created or the effect you have had on others. As you bring back your breath at the end of the evening, identify three positives in your life. Breathe in while focusing on the first positive, and breathe out while releasing the gray, foggy fear.

Examples of three positives in your life could be three qualities in your spouse you took for granted this week, three ways you've had a positive influence on another person's life, or even three people, places, or things that make you smile, including the guy at the office whose jokes are terrible but still make you laugh. With each inhale, bring the positive into full focus, seeing all the good until you find yourself able to smile during the bad. Just a few minutes of reminding yourself of how much you truly have will not only change your internal monitor of success but also bring you to a place of much-needed rest.

Light Clearing

You are among the fortunate if you have had a stress-free day. These are the days you take the scenic route home with the windows down and a breeze in your hair. We long for these days, but for the high-octane human, they are rare. Clearing is still an essential part of your evening, but on the really good days, instead of spending time removing the thick layers of today's build-up, your time is spent setting intentions for a great tomorrow and a restful sleep. Like with MM#5, gratitude is the key to a successful light clearing. As you bring back your breath, bring back the gratitude, for today's triumphs deserve to be acknowledged. If you can clearly see the great things the universe is doing in your life today, reconnect stress-free and watch gratitude lift you up to become an even greater person. Smile as you lay your head on your pillow of peace, for today has been a good day! Slowly count your successes instead of sheep.

When you are engaged in life and open to opportunities each day, the exciting as well as the unexpected (both good and bad) are part of a regular day. The new people and events that yesterday you could not have imagined are now part of today's normal. As you enter a clearing at the end of the day, whether heavy or light, allow an anticipation for tomorrow's possibilities bring a smile as you drift off to sleep. Sure, the past still exists in the back of your mind, but it no longer controls you when kept where it belongs—in the past.

As you become a master of *Six Small Meditation Meals a Day*, you enter the evening with less build up leading to more nights of light clearing than heavy in the same way that eating smaller meals during the day helps you avoid a heavy meal at night brought on by skipping meals during the active part of your day. We all know the heavy feeling of the bulging buffet when eaten in the evening. By not skipping MM#1–MM#5, you help to bring lightness to MM#6, which leads to a more restful sleep, less anxiety, and the sweetest of dreams.

Here's the Heart of a Heavy Clearing: Eight Minutes

Begin by visualizing a soft blue pillow of air as you breathe in, choosing one of the three strategies (or all of them) based of what your body needs. Hold the blue air in and breathe out the gray, dusty fog, sending all the build-up along with it. Be specific to yourself about who or what needs to leave your head. The negativity that may have caused you stress today does not define you; it defines the ones causing you frustration. Keep them out of your head as you drift off to sleep and remember how far you've come in your life. Repeat this process until you feel the outer crusty layer being peeled away.

Here's the Skinny on a Light Clearing: Eight Minutes

Begin by visualizing the stars at night over the calming waves of the ocean or with the sound of a mountain stream. Breathe in, smile, and be grateful for today's successes. Hold for seven seconds and breathe out. Breathe in gratitude with each new breath. Continue as you drift off to sleep.

NOTIFICATIONS
THAT NOURISH

Replacing one large meditation meal with six mini-meals is the key to making the most of the benefits of meditation. Just by reading this book, you are on your way to taking back your day by controlling the way you react to stress. In the early morning hours with MM#1, you bring clarity to your thoughts and create a fresh energy with which to start your day. You make connections that remind you all is well and tap into your intuition where new thoughts are waiting to move you to greater outcomes today.

By mid-morning at MM#2, you create an immunity to workplace stress by giving yourself permission to focus on this morning only and choosing to react as your soul-self and not your ego-self. As you strap on your blinders, you give respect to the people and events that need your full attention this very morning.

Lunchtime brings time to be inspired and draw in much-needed creative time for yourself that naturally leads to inspiring others. MM#3 becomes a treasured span of guilt-free inspiration you look forward to daily. By 4 p.m., workday stress demands you step outside your limited view with MM#4 and see a much larger life picture. Your pelican perspective brings you to a place of fresh understanding in the afternoon when energy dwindles and mindsets narrow.

MM#5 is a welcome and refreshing evening meditation that focuses on being good to yourself and reconnecting with your passions. A little gratitude will go a long way in this mini-meditation.

As you end your day, the ever-important MM#6 allows you to clear the crust, whether heavy or light, finding your breath one last time today as you prepare for sleep. Learning how to push away the negative before bedtime and remind yourself how far you have come helps send you off to a night of restful peace.

Even on the really good days, it is important not to skip the mini-meditation meals. The focus may change, but the internal routine remains in place allowing the universe at least six times a day to do its work on you. While you are busy connecting with the universe, it is a good idea to connect your mini-meditation meals to an app on your personal phone or computer with habit reminders to keep track of your progress and send you notifications for each meditation. Unlike the many notifications already pulling for your attention each day, make these notifications unique and soothing.

Like Pavlov's dogs, we jump, react, and ignore all in the name of notifications. Words like *Aurora*, *Calypso*, and *Swish* are too familiar to us. We react one way for an email notification, another way for a breaking news story, and we rarely miss a social media post of extreme insignificance. Your body sends you notifications every time it is out of sync from workday stress—and yet, we ignore those notifications completely.

By connecting all six meditation meals to an app with habit reminders, you are able to receive gentle but consistent encouragement that brings a much-needed sense of peace. Unlike the notifications that send us plundering under papers and through purses for our mighty cell phones, these meditation reminders should be distinct and cause you to smile when heard amid the chaos of work, budget dilemmas, or even while in a client meeting. Instead of turning the phone off when stressed, use it to remind you and nourish you by keeping track of your progress toward a better you!

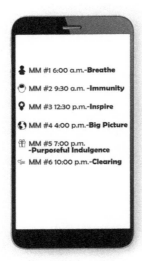

Figure 1: My phone with habit reminders and custom icons. I use the Productive-Habit Tracker (available for iPhone) as I found it worked the best with what I was trying to accomplish.

DAYDREAMS AND LOTTERY TICKETS

As the sun blankets my entire body, I can see the boats in the distance pulling into the harbor, reminding me of the fresh seafood this island is known for. The clear, blue water and salty air ease me to a place of much-needed peace and quiet. *Crap! The reports are due in ten minutes. Where have I been and where did the time go? Who turned up the heat in this office?*

You are busy, engaged, and motivated, but it is easy to get distracted in today's world. Even with a routine in place full of reminders and notifications drawing you back to a place of inner understanding, we still let scattered thoughts cloud our day. For the busy human, adding six moments throughout your day may seem impossible, but when you eliminate the minutes of extraneous thinking, you are not adding more time. Instead, you are using the time in a more productive way. We use daydreams to relieve stress, a defense mechanism to the mounting aggravations of work or home. Yet the result leaves us feeling farther behind, and more frustration follows.

In business, daydreams can be the cloud within which new ideas have taken shape in the pre-implementation phase, but they also pull us away from the dedicated focus for today. It is easy to spend forty-five meaningless minutes a day thinking about how we would spend the proceeds of a winning lottery ticket. Now imagine replacing that forty-five minutes with time purely focused on something with much better odds for your future: ten minutes inspiring yourself through an online course or ten minutes of creative time (MM#3), fifteen minutes in genuine self-care with gratitude (MM#5), or eight minutes making sure you are not bringing baggage to bed with you (MM#6). Changing the way you spend your thinking time will change the way you think.

Some of the top CEOs of some of the world's most successful businesses have admitted to having ADHD. In fact, issues with distraction are common among entrepreneurs and Type A personalities. These masters of multitasking are successful in part because they use their ADHD as a strength instead of a hinderance. Six meditation meals a day help turn distraction into increased moments of clarity by providing scheduled, focused breaks throughout the day. For the highly distracted, these six moments of clarity increase attention far greater than any Adderall could ever do.

Six meditation meals act as a tool that brings you back to a place of peace in a way that dreaming of a salty lounge chair never will (unless of course, you are actually in that chair!). These six mini-meditations when paired with gentle notifications pull you out of cloudy distraction and daydreams and bring you to a place of progress in your day. Unlike scattered thoughts that leave you feeling guilty and less effective, the six focus times throughout the day become a guilt-free span of stress release. When you are more in touch with yourself through meditation, the daydreaming is needed less and as it fades, it is replaced with focused, creative moments that lead to success in your home life, a feeling of being ahead of schedule, and increased odds that far outweigh your chances of winning big at the gas station.

TO BEACH OR NOT
TO BEACH

Before meditation became a household word, stress relief from work came in many forms: a run through the park, a few drinks after work, or falling asleep in front of the TV thirty minutes after getting home. The weekend turns into the opposite of the focused diligence at the office—late night partying, binge-eating, and napping all day Sunday, the things that leave you feeling nothing but hungover and dreading the Monday drive to work. When not treated, this buildup of stress can turn your long-anticipated vacation into a long stretch of catch-up. For many, that means catching up on sleep, finally reading that book sitting on your nightstand, or cramming in everything you have been missing into one week of paid vacation.

On vacation, *routine* brain is traded for completely *free* brain, but sadly, routine brain comes back with a vengeance after your week at the beach. Ever notice how packing is so much more fun than unpacking, or the energy you have in anticipation of this freedom is so much greater than the lack of energy piling in your laundry room after the break?

Meditation came along and changed everything. Keep in mind, meditation trains the brain and with a little practice implementing six small meditations throughout the day, routine brain is switched out permanently for a free and aware brain that sees a bigger picture and allows thoughts to be clear and full of gratitude.

Now that your brain has changed the way you handle workday stress changes, and with six mini-meditations in place, the stress is less—and what used to aggravate you suddenly doesn't bother you at all. Time to decompress becomes less urgent, and your spa-like attitude carries you through even the roughest of weeks. With stress under control, the weekend goes from Goody's extra-strength to a relaxing and meaningful time away from the office.

Vacation also takes on a whole new meaning. Having mastered the workday stress, vacation goes from concentrated time to catch up and decompress to time spent the way it was meant to be: time simply spent. Whether spent in pursuit of new experiences or pouring time into family, the off-work hours and especially vacation take on a whole new energy. Instead of living for the breaks from work, you begin living fully each day. With life in balance, we are now equipped to exist in a place of joy when there is no vacation at all.

Quitting a secure job to start your own business or running a family-owned business can mean sacrifice when it comes to vacation. Six meditation meals bring strength on the home-front by having you turn inward for sustenance. As we form meditative habits that develop into second nature practices throughout the workday, we create our own happy place no matter where we are! Keep the success and leave behind the stress.

CONCLUSION

I used to think that if I could only get through this one graduate course or this one busy season of work, then the stress would change. If I could get to a better financial place, or find the perfect employee, then the stress would change. The truth is that as soon as one stressor leaves, new stress finds its way in. The fact is, stress and the lessons associated with it never end. But the good news is that by changing the way you view the stress in your life, you empower yourself to conquer the stress and not let it control your life like before. As you allow six meditation meals to change you from the inside out, the changes you will see in your life reach far beyond the office.

In fact, the implications of workday meditations are so far-reaching that they may even surprise you and the people around you.

Renewed Relationships

Of the six small meditations a day, the one that has had the greatest impact on my personal relationships has been MM#4—*Big Picture*. Having a big picture mentality at work where struggles are lessons allowed me to see how key people in my life outside of work are perfectly placed in my life for a reason. Life lessons have been and will continue to challenge you no matter where you are, and simply seeing others in your life as part of your divine journey takes away the friction and frustration that can come from the people we are closest to.

Think of three big lessons you have learned in life so far. Now think of the people who have helped make your lessons possible. If your lesson involves being a better father, you are likely to have at least one challenging kid. If your lesson is being more understanding of an opinion that is very different from yours, don't be surprised when one of your siblings goes off in an unexpected direction. Just one teenager alone can teach you patience, unconditional love, and understanding different viewpoints *all* in the first summer he or she turns sixteen. Even your ex, whom an outsider might view as a major mistake, can now be seen as a necessary part of a perfect journey to the best you!

Seeing life differently through six meditation meals a day allows you to see the people in your life differently, too. By turning inward six times each day, a new person in you emerges, and suddenly life and the people in your life make sense. You will go from taking these people for granted to taking them to a place of new respect as you see them as part of this well-designed journey known as your life.

The teacher who used to come home every afternoon frustrated with high school freshmen now greets her husband at the door with a refreshing smile instead of dumping the drama onto him the moment he pulls into the driveway. The now-mindful college student who used to ignore classmates different from him in high school now creates a lasting friendship with his randomly placed and very different roommate. Honor those people the universe has led into your life, for they are an important part of your personal journey.

Here's to Your Health
I mentioned earlier in the book that mini-meditations throughout the day began for me as a way to address the stress before completely falling apart. Migraines were causing me to miss work and social opportunities. Sleepless nights showered me with bad dreams and made my mornings feel listless and foggy. Frequent sore throats and doctor visits were frustrating, and the costly MRIs and false alarms leading to more doctor visits were relentless. I remember being referred to the best gastroenterologist in Charlotte, and after weeks of waiting for an appointment and hours of waiting in the office in pain, I was told there was nothing wrong with me.

I should have jumped for joy, but when you realize now that it's just the *stress* causing your gut to be tied in knots, what do you do? I was desperate for a solution and somehow knew medication was not the answer. Instead, I turned to meditation. Morning-based meditation practices that became popular among thousands of people were a great starting place and a great help but just not enough to keep me going all day.

By breaking up my day with mini-meditations the way I was spreading out my meals, I was able to get away from one larger meditation once a day with effects that had faded by lunchtime. As the mini-meditations became routine, major changes began to happen in my medical chart. In fact, since beginning six meditation meals a day, my chart is empty, and my doctors' names don't roll off my tongue anymore. It feels great to be set free from migraines and sore throats and to feel rested in the morning.

Imagine the success once you eliminate the stress! You are now clear and focused in the morning, you are grounded and not thrown off by the aggravations of mid-morning, and you've found a way to work in creative time daily. Your struggles take on new meaning as life lessons and a big picture attitude creates renewed relationships in your life where your closest people are valued and not taken for granted. You are taking care of yourself, sleeping better, and, best of all, you feel great! By taking back your day in a meditative way, you find the person you were always meant to be, and you will love the person you become—the person who is slow to anger and open to new perspectives. The person who has great ideas on a Tuesday and knows when to keep ego out of the picture, making you the perfect blend of boss and Buddha!

Being aware of how you spend your thinking time makes the most of your moments. As you look back over your life, you can see what has brought you to where you are today, which didn't happen in one giant event but instead can be found in the mini moments. Those moments you didn't think much of at the time have created the person you are today. As you turn inward through six meditation meals a day, your moments will now have purpose, and the masterpiece that is your life will be amazing! Make these moments count.

CPSIA information can be obtained
at www.ICGtesting.com
Printed in the USA
LVHW091418220819
628593LV00001B/184/P

9 781733 897396